ESSENTIALLY YOURS

Aromatherapy
Pocket Guide

Susan Anderson
Seeds for Change Wellness

First Printing, 2016

Seeds for Change Wellness
105 Oak Drive
Sellersville, PA 18960

www.seedsforchangewellness.com
https://www.facebook.com/Seeds-for-Change-Wellness

DISCLAIMER

This pocket guide is a reference work and is not intended to treat, diagnose, or prescribe. The information presented here is in no way to be considered as a substitute for consultation and treatment with a licensed healthcare professional.

Essential Oils (EO's), like medications, may be harmful and dangerous if used improperly. In order to obtain the full therapeutic benefits from EOs it is important to know how to use them correctly. EOs are highly concentrated forms of aromatic energy, with some having a low therapeutic margin. Choosing the correct method of application, knowing the correct dosages, and being aware of contra-indications are important factors, ensuring safe and responsible use. Careful consideration and assessment needs to be made when determining the dosage amounts for all individuals, in particular the dosage adjustments required for the frail, the elderly and children.

Some EOs can be taken internally, **but this is recommended for only the safest oils, at the correct dosage level**. Many who practice therapeutic application of EOs feel this method should only be used by medical doctors. This is my position as well. *I do not recommend nor do I practice internal application of EOs.* A condition can be treated effectively and safely when the above criteria-- of selection, administration methods, and proper dosage amounts is followed.

Susan Anderson
Seeds for Change Wellness

TABLE OF CONTENTS

INTRODUCTION

Aromatherapy is a wonderful tool to have in your toolbox when choosing to follow a healthy, natural life style.

Aromatherapy is the use of essential oils, applied through either inhaling or applying directly to the body, in order to restore and balance oneself on all levels- physically, mentally, emotionally and spiritually. Truly a holistic approach to self-care!

The essential oils are extracted from natural plant material such as the flower, seeds, bark, root, resin, and leaves of plants, to name a few. These essential oils are powerful healers, and are better suited for helping to restore balance within the body than their synthetic counterparts. A guiding principle of use is to stimulate and strengthen our immune system so it begins the self-healing process.

Although Aromatherapy has ancient roots, it has been enjoying a modern day resurgence, with many choosing to learn how to incorporate essential oils into their daily lives.

Just like anything else, individual results may vary. Many factors need to be considered when assessing the effectiveness of a selected essential oil for a particular individual. What is our state of mind at the time? Is what we are dealing with an acute or chronic situation? Is there more than one imbalance needing immediate attention? What is the underlying root cause? Each individual brings their own set of circumstance to the table, so it is understandable that results may vary from person to person.

When we have been diagnosed with an illness, it did not just present itself at the time of diagnosis, but has most likely been years in the making. We get so used to instant gratification and results and expect the same thing with our body, mind and spirit But just as it was a process over time for an imbalance to present itself, it may be the same lengthy process to reverse it and get to that root cause so a healing can occur. We must be patient and be willing to do the work required.

For those who are interested in dipping their toes in and learning about how to incorporate Aromatherapy into their daily routine, the amount of information can be overwhelming!

The purpose of this book is to learn how to effectively and safely introduce a measured use of essential oils into your life. You will learn the foundations to get started with emphasis placed upon what I consider to be the 5 best essential oils to have in your holistic medicine cabinet as well as for personal care and household use.

Take your time & enjoy the journey!

WHAT IS AROMATHERAPY?

Aromatherapy means the use of aromas for their healing properties. Restoration of physical, mental, emotional and spiritual health, through the application of essential oils can also be called Holistic Aromatherapy.

THE BASICS: UNDERSTANDING ESSENTIAL OILS
The term essential is applied to these oils because they contain the essence or fragrant part of the plant. They can be referred to as the "life blood" of the plant.

ALL ESSENTIAL OILS ARE VOLATILE
They evaporate when exposed to air, even at normal room temperatures and become vapor. Rates of evaporation vary among essential oils.

ESSENTIAL OILS ARE NOT OILY
Oils such as almond, canola, safflower, and peanut are fixed or carrier oils and are very different from essential oils. The base or carrier oils feel oily to the touch, and when exposed to air become rancid and do not evaporate.

Essential oils are not oily, do not leave an oily residue, do not become rancid and they evaporate readily.

PURE VS SYNTHETIC
Pure essential oils come from plants and have an extremely complex chemical structure. Synthetic oils are chemical replicas of essential oils and lack a life force.

WHERE ARE ESSENTIAL OILS FOUND?
Essential oils are found in various parts of plants, as indicated in the list below:

ESSENTIAL OIL/PLANT SOURCE

Valerian- Root
Cinnamon- Bark
Juniper: Berry
Nutmeg- Nut
Benzoin – Resin
Lavender- Flower
Peppermint- Leaf
Fir- Needle
Garlic- Bulbs
Fennel- Seeds
Bergamot- Fruit Peel

PURCHASING ESSENTIAL OILS

* Buy your oils from a reputable company
* Purchase only 100% pure and natural, not synthetic oils
* Be sure it is listed by its Latin name
* Do the sniff test- you can tell a lot about quality

RECOMMENDED COMPANIES

* Aura Cacia
* Frontier
* Mountain Rose Herbs
* NOW
* Young Living

STORAGE

* Store in a cool dark place away from direct sunlight
* Store in glass not plastic whenever possible
* Keep away from homeopathic remedies- they will antidote
  the remedy
* Keep from oxidizing

THERAPEUTIC PROPERTIES

There are many therapeutic values associated with the various essential oils. A short list includes: antibacterial, antifungal, antiviral, anti-inflammatory, antidepressant, antiseptic, digestive, decongestant, stimulant, and tonic.

WHERE TO START

This book covers information on 5 basic essential oils that are a good jumping off point to introduce yourself to the benefits of using essential oils in your daily life. These 5 are very practical to have on hand for your home medicine chest, personal care and household needs. Covered will be: Lavender, Eucalyptus, Rosemary, Peppermint, and Tea Tree.

Take your time and become familiar with each of these essential oils. Learn their therapeutic properties, what part of the plant they come from, what they smell like, as well as when and how to use them. Once you have done this, then begin to add new essential oils to your list.

Why? When we try to learn too much too quickly, things can get jumbled. We may get confused or frustrated, then what started out as a true desire to learn might be set aside or discarded. My intent is to have you take this journey in measured steps, so it has a greater chance of becoming integrated into your daily life.

METHODS OF APPLICATION

In order to obtain the full therapeutic benefits from essential oils it is important to know how to use them correctly. Essential oils are highly concentrated forms of aromatic energy, with some having a low therapeutic margin. Choosing the correct method of application, knowing the correct dosage, and being aware of contra-indications are important factors, ensuring safe and responsible use.

FULL BATH
Run bath, then add essential oil, close the bathroom door so vapors do not escape. Dosage: As indicated for external dosage for the selected EO

SITZ BATH
Run bath to hip level or use a bowl large enough to fit your behind into, add EO, swish thoroughly to disperse. Dosage: 2-3 drops

HAND BATH
Fill bowl with warm water, add EO, mix to disperse, soak hands for about 10 minutes. Dosage: 2-4 drops

FOOT BATH
Fill pan or container with warm to hot water, add EO, mix to disperse, soak feet for 15-20 minutes. Dosage: 2-4 drops

MASSAGE OIL
Select a base or carrier oil that is best for the purpose of the massage. Use a carrier that is cold pressed. Never use lanolin or mineral oil as a base. Add the selected EO. Shake well to blend. If you are creating a synergy, blend the EOs first, shaking several minutes, then add the carrier oil. Dosage: 5 drops per tsp of carrier oil

COMPRESSES

A hot or cold compress can be made depending on the situation. A hot compress is made with boiling water, a cold compress with ice water. Add EO to the water. Place the material being used for the compress into the water (unbleached muslin is a good choice) wring out, then apply to the affected area. <u>Dosage</u>: 6 drops to 9 oz. of water

CREAMS/LOTIONS

For some conditions it is effective to add EO to a base cream or lotion. The cream or lotion should be unscented and lanolin free, made from plant products. Lotions are good for covering large areas of the body. A small amount of jojoba or avocado oil added to the lotion will help keep it from dragging on the skin and makes it a more nourishing blend. Creams are ideal for skin problems such as rashes, athlete's foot, eczema and psoriasis. <u>Dosage:</u> Variable, check the requirements for the selected EO's

INHALED AS A VAPOR

Pour hot water into a bowl, add EO. Cover head with a towel, lean over bowl, keep face 10" away. Breathe deeply through nose. Can also be used in a vaporizer, keep dosages the same. <u>Dosage</u>: 2-3 drops, duration 5 minutes

INHALED USING A TISSUE

Put EO on a tissue or handkerchief, inhale deeply through the nose. <u>Dosage:</u> 1 drop, duration as needed

INHALED AS A NASAL SPRAY

Add EO to carrier oil. Blend well. <u>Dosage:</u> EO 2 drops per TBS of carrier oil, duration as needed

NASAL INHALER

Fill a small glass bottle with sea salt. Add EO. Shake well to disperse EO. <u>Dosage</u>: EO 1-2 drops, duration inhale as needed

SUPPOSITORIES
Mix EO with cocoa butter. Powdered herbs can also be added for additional therapeutic effect. <u>Dosage</u>: EO: 6 drops per 2 TBS of cocoa butter

AEROSOL AIR DISPERSION
Room sprays can be made as an effective method of dispersing EO into the air. Fill a spray bottle with warm distilled water. Add EO. Shake vigorously to blend. Shake well again before each use. Use as you would an air freshener. <u>Dosage</u>: This will vary depending on the formula followed or created. A general rule is 6 drops EO for each cup of water

DOUCHE
Add EO to a pint of warm water. Shake well. <u>Dosage</u>: Check dosage amount for selected EO

HUMIDIFERS
Add EO to water in humidifier. <u>Dosage</u>: EO 2-3 drops

LIGHT BULBS
Add EO to a light bulb ring that can be placed on top of the bulb. When the light is turned on, it will disperse the EO into the air. <u>Dosage</u>: EO 1-2 drops

OINTMENTS/SALVES
Ointments may be a more suitable carrier for certain conditions, such as in treatment of cuts, scrapes and wounds than a vegetable oil base. A general formula is 4 TBS anhydrous lanolin and 2 TBS almond oil which is blended together in a double boiler. When well blended together and cooled, add the EO. A stiffer base can be made by adding a ½ oz of grated beeswax during the double boiling stage. <u>Dosage</u>: 5 drops EO per carrier base

FLORAL WATER

A floral water can be made with EO to be used as a body spray or splash. Add the EO to distilled water and shake well before using. I also add a few drops of castor oil to help disperse the EO. Dosage: 3 drops EO to 4 oz. of distilled water

PERFUME

A perfume blend can be made using EO. One should strive to create a balancing, fragrant blend of aromas. This can be achieved by experimenting with blends of EOs. A standard formula should include a top note, a middle note and a base note EO. Once the EOs are selected, place them in a clean, sterilized dark bottle and shake well for several minutes to create the synergy. In a perfume it is a good practice to allow the synergistic blend to age for several weeks, shaking the blend daily in the initial stages. Once you have aged your blend, then add the carrier. This could be grain alcohol or vegetable glycerin. Dosage: Create a synergistic blend totaling 20 drops of EO to each ounce of carrier oil. A blending formula could be: Top Note: 10 drops, Mid Note: 7 drops, Base Note: 3 drops

MAY CAUSE SKIN IRRITATION

Almond Bitter **
Allspice
Anise
Basil
Benzoin Resinoid
Bergamot
Black Pepper
Cajuput
Camphor **
Cedarwood
Chamomile
Cinnamon
Clove Leaf
Dill
Eucalyptus
Fennel
Garlic
Ginger
Grapefruit
Lemon
Lemon Balm
Parsley
Peppermint
Pine
Spearmint
Thyme

** Avoid Using

SKIN PATCH TEST

A skin Patch Test can be used to test sensitivity to an EO. Dermal irritation may occur if an oil is administered incorrectly in too high a concentration when applied externally or if you have sensitive skin or allergies

PERFORMING A SKIN PATCH TEST

Clean an area on your forearm and dry it thoroughly. Apply a drop of the EO being tested to that spot on the arm. Wait 24 hours, then check the area tested. If no reaction has occurred, then you passed the test!

If there is any indication of a sensitivity or reaction, it will appear as a red spot, itching or blistering. If that is the case, then the oil needs to be diluted or should be omitted and substituted for another oil.

When using EOs it is important to adhere to the recommended dosages because of their potency and to keep in mind that the therapeutic margin can be low for some oils.

If you have particularly sensitive skin, it may be best to conduct this test with the EO diluted in a bland base oil and then apply this dilution to the arm.

DO NOT USE DURING PREGNANCY

Almond Bitter **
Anise
Basil
Bay Leaf
Birch
Black Pepper
Camphor **
Cedarwood
Celery Seed
Chamomile *
Cinnamon
Citronella
Clary Sage
Clove Leaf/Bud
Cypress
Elecampane
Elemi
Fennel
Garlic
Geranium *
Ginger
Hyssop
Immortelle
Juniper
Lemon Balm
Marjoram
Mugwort
Myrrh
Nutmeg
Oregano
Parsley
Pennyroyal
Peppermint *
Pine
Rose Attar *

Rosemary *
Rue
Sage
Sassafras
Tansy
Tea Tree
Thyme
Thuja
Wintergreen
Ylang Ylang

** Avoid using in aromatherapy

*   Indicated not to be used during First Trimester.

 Unless you have a good understanding of aromatherapy it is better to avoid its use when pregnant

CARRIER OIL REFERENCE

A carrier oil is just what it says, it holds or carries the essential oils. Remember essential oils are, with a few exceptions, always diluted. Below are some of the choices you can select from.

ALMOND OIL is mildly pale, with a light floral scent. Advantages: An emollient, nourishing to skin, used as a base in many beauty products (creams), closest to our natural skin oils, helps relieve itching, soreness, dryness, blends well with EOs. Disadvantages: Leaves oily coating on skin, must be protected from light and heat.

AVOCADO OIL is nutty tasting, pale green with a strong earthy aroma. Advantages: Is penetrating, spreads easily, excellent moisturizer, helpful for dry and aging skin, helpful in treating slow to heal sores and eczema, used in beauty products (cosmetics, soaps). Disadvantages: Becomes cloudy if chilled, needs to be added last to retain vitamins.

CALENDULA INFUSED OIL is golden yellow in color with a floral taste and aroma. Advantages: Contains vitamin A and carotene, good for maintaining healthy skin, has astringent properties, detoxifying, anti-inflammatory, anti-infectious, beneficial for use in healing wounds. Disadvantages: Expensive to purchase but can be made easily from fresh or dried organically grown Calendula officinalis flowers.

GRAPESEED OIL is light, colorless, and slightly sweet tasting. Advantages: Absorbs quickly into the skin, beneficial for acne or oily skin types, mildly astringent. Disadvantages: Will leave an oily residue on the body, is polyunsaturated making it unstable and needs to be protected from sunlight and heat.

JOJOBA OIL is a wax rather than an oil, is golden yellow in color, has a waxy taste and aroma. <u>Advantages</u>: Quickly absorbs into the skin, spreads easily without leaving a shine, good for all skin types, especially beneficial for aging skin, similar to sebum produced by our skin, very stable lasts for extended periods of time. <u>Disadvantages</u>: Very heavy, best used as a blend with other carriers.

OLIVE OIL is faint tasting, pale yellow or greenish oil with a heavy olive scent. <u>Advantages</u>: Nourishing and soothing to skin, helpful in softening hard skin or inflamed areas, useful for eczema and psoriasis, frequently used as a base for massage or bath oils, used in making ointments, cheaper substitute for sweet-almond oil. <u>Disadvantages</u>: Leaves a heavy oily coating on skin, needs protection from light, becomes cloudy at cool temperatures, can have an over powering aroma if not diluted.

PEANUT OIL is bland tasting, pale yellow with a light nutty scent. <u>Advantages</u>: Used in products for dry skin (soaps, creams) helpful in massage oil for muscle and joint conditions (arthritis/rheumatism) a cheaper substitute for sweet almond oil. <u>Disadvantages</u>: Leaves an oily coating on the skin, needs protection from light, becomes cloudy at cool room temperatures, has a low shelf life.

SESAME OIL has a pale yellow color, which has a strong sesame odor if unrefined, nutty taste. <u>Advantages</u>: Top quality lubricant for rheumatic conditions, is a natural skin cleanser, useful for psoriasis, dry skin and eczema, contains a natural preservative and is more stable than most oils. <u>Disadvantages</u>: Leaves a somewhat oily coating on the skin.

SUNFLOWER OIL has a slight aroma, and a clear, pale yellow color. <u>Advantages</u>: Leaves skin smooth and non greasy, effective for external ulcers, bruises and dermatitis, is native to the US, no pesticides are used in the growing process. <u>Disadvantages</u>: Needs to be protected from light.

WHEAT GERM OIL is a thick oil with a nutty aroma, is orange to yellow color, with a nutty taste. <u>Advantages:</u> Excellent source of Vitamin E, good for the skin, helpful in speeding up the healing of cuts and wounds, effective in preventing and reducing scarring. Provides anti-oxidant action when added to massage and bath oil blends to preserve their properties. <u>Disadvantages</u>: Needs to be kept away from direct light, thick and heavy when applied to the skin.

SAFE FOR UNDILUTED APPLICATION

Generally, as a rule essential oils should not be used undiluted or neat on the skin. There are a few that are viewed as safe. These include:

Lavender: *Lavandula angustifolia*
Tea Tree: *Melaleuca alternifolia*
Helichrysum*: Helichrysum italicum*
Chamomile: *Chamaemelum nobile*

WHEN TO USE UNDILUTED ON SKIN

Spot treatment of acne
Cold Sore
Minor Burn
Bug Bites
Headaches
Reflex Work/Acupressure/Acupuncture
Minor bruises/skin trauma

Phototoxic Reactions

Some essential oils cause a phototoxic reaction, meaning they may cause a skin irritation when applied to skin that is exposed to the sun. When applied, dermatitis may occur.

PHOTOXIC REACTIONS MAY INCLUDE

Blistering
Changes in skin color
Rash
Severe sunburn
Swelling

ESSENTIAL OILS IN THE CITRUS family are known to be phototoxic. These include:

Bergamot: *Citrus bergamia*
Bitter Orange: *Citrus aurantium*
Grapefruit: *Citrus paradisi*
Lime: *Citrus medica*
Sweet Orange: *Citrus sinensis*
Lemon: *Citrus limon*
Mandarin: *Citrus reticulata*

If using any of these essential oils, avoid exposure to ultra violet rays for at least 12- 18 hours.

THERAPEUTIC PROPERTIES GLOSSARY

ALTERNATIVE: Actions that slowly and positively "alter" the condition of the body by purifying the blood. They help the body to assimilate nutrients and eliminate waste products of metabolism.

ANALGESIC: Anything given to reduce pain without resulting in loss of consciousness

ANTIBACTERIAL: Actions that can prevent bacterial growth.

ANTIBIOTIC: Actions that destroy or arrest growth of harmful micro-organisms

ANTIOXIDANT: Any substance that reduces damage due to oxygen

ANTISEPTIC: A substance that kills or prevents the growth of bacteria

ASTRIGENT: Actions that have a binding/constricting effect (shrinks blood vessels) and can reduce secretions and discharges. (Most of these contain tannic acid.)

BITTERS: Stimulate the appetite and the release of digestive juices.

CARMINATIVE: Actions that sooth the digestive tract and relieve gas and bowel cramps

DIAPHORETIC: A substance that promotes sweating

DIURETIC: A substance that encourages urination

EMETIC: Promotes vomiting

EMMENAGOGUE: Promotes menstruation

EXPECTORANT: A substance that promotes the secretion or expulsion of phlegm, mucus, or other matter from the respiratory tract.

FEBRIFUGE: Reduces a fever

NERVINE: Having a soothing calming effect on the nerves

RUBEFACIENT: Produces redness of the skin, increases circulation

STYPTIC: Stops bleeding

TONIC: Actions that strengthen or invigorate organs or the entire body

VERMIFUGE: Actions that expel worms/parasites

VULNERARY: Actions that heal wounds by promoting cell growth and repair

DILUTING ESSENTIAL OILS

Essential oils are meant to be diluted in almost all cases. Use the information below when diluting your essential oils.

DILUTION RATES

FOR CHILDREN
25% Rate
Avoid using with children under 2 years of age
1 drop per 4 TSP carrier oil

FRAIL/ELDERLY/SICK ADULTS
1% Rate
1 drop per TSP
5-6 drop per ounce

ADULTS
2% Rate
2 drops per TSP
10 -12 drops per ounce

MEASUREMENT EQUIVALENCES

100 drops= 1 tsp = 5ml = 1/6 ounce
200 drops = 2 tsp = 10ml = 1/3 ounce
300 drops = 3 tsp = 15ml = 1/2 ounce
400 drops = 4 tsp = 20ml = 2/3 ounce
500 drops = 5 tsp = 25ml = 5/6 ounce
600 drops = 6 tsp = 30ml = 1 ounce

CATEGORIES & NOTES

Essential oils are classified by their scents, into categories and notes. Notes are broken into 3 areas: top notes, middle notes, and base notes.

CLASSIFICATION CATEGORIES

FLORAL: Examples: Lavender, Rose, Jasmine
WOODSY: Examples: Pine, Sandalwood, Cedar
EARTHY: Examples: Patchouli, Vetiver
HERBACEOUS: Examples: Basil, Rosemary
MINTY: Examples: Peppermint, Spearmint
CAMPHORACEOUS: Examples: Eucalyptus, Tea Tree
SPICY: Examples: Clove, Cinnamon, Ginger
CITRUS: Examples: Orange, Bergamo, Grapefruit

BLEND WELL TOGETHER:

FLORAL blends with woodsy, spicy, citrus
WOODSY blends with: all
EARTHY blends with woodsy, minty
HERBACEOUS blends with woodsy, minty
MINTY blends with woodsy, earthy, herbaceous, citrus
CAMPHORACEOUS blends with woodsy
SPICY blends with floral, woodsy, citrus
CITRUS blends with woodsy, minty, spicy

ESSENTIAL OIL NOTES

The "note" of an essential oil blend is how quickly it evaporates. When you put a blend of essential oils on your skin it will smell one way, but 3 hours later it may smell another way, because some of the oils in your blend have evaporated. These notes are based on the musical scale and are referred to as top notes, middle notes, and base notes.

TOP NOTES
* Evaporate very quickly
* Tend to be light, refreshing, and uplifting
* Usually inexpensive in price
* Very volatile
* Give the first impression from a blend
* 10 -30 Percent of a blend

MIDDLE NOTES
* Most essential oils fall into this category
* Gives body to a blend, known as the heart of a blend
* Have a balancing effect
* Tend to be warm and soft scents
* Not apparent at first
* 30 to 60 percent of a blend

BASE NOTES
* Are the foundation of a blend
* Are heavy, deep, penetrating
* Last a long time, evaporate slowly
* Gives a blend its staying power
* Tend to be the most expensive essential oils
* 15- 30 percent of a blend

CATEGORIES EXPANDED LIST

These are the main categories of classification, some essential oils can appear under more than one classification.

FLORAL
Chamomile
Geranium
Jasmine
Lavender
Neroli
Rose
Ylang Ylang

WOODSY
Cedarwood
Cinnamon
Cypress
Juniper Berry
Pine
Sandalwood

HERBACEOUS
Basil
Clary Sage
Hyssop
Marjoram
Melissa
Rosemary

MINTY
Peppermint
Spearmint

EARTHY
Angelica
Patchouli
Valerian
Vetiver

CAMPHORACEOUS
Cajuput
Eucalyptus
Rosemary
Tea Tree

SPICY
Black Pepper
Cardamom
Cinnamon
Coriander
Cumin
Ginger
Nutmeg

CITRUS
Bergamot
Grapefruit
Lemon
Lime
Orange
Tangerine

RESINOUS
Benzoin
Elemi
Frankincense
Myrrh

TOP * MIDDLE * BASE NOTES EXPANDED LIST

TOP NOTES

Anise
Basil
Bay Laurel
Bergamot
Citronella
Eucalyptus
Galbanum
Grapefruit
Lavender
Lavendin

Lemon
Lemongrass
Lime
Orange
Peppermint
Petitgrain
Spearmint
Tagets
Tangerine

MIDDLE NOTES

Bay
Cajeput
Carrot Seed
Chamomile
Cinnamon
Clary Sage
Clove Bud
Cypress
Dill
Elemi
Fennel
Fir Needle
Geranium
Hyssop
Jasmine
Juniper Berry
Marjoram

Neroli
Palmarosa
Parsley
Pepper, Black
Pine
Rose
Rose Geranium
Rosemary
Rosewood
Spruce
Tea Tree
Thyme
Yarrow
Ylang Ylang

BASE NOTES

Angelica
Balsam
Benzoin
Cedarwood
Frankincense
Ginger
Helichrysum
Myrrh
Oakmoss
Patchouli
Sandalwood
Vanilla
Vetiver

LET'S BEGIN!

5 STARTER OILS

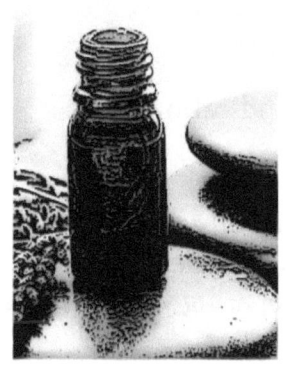

FIVE BASIC ESSENTIAL OILS

This next section gives you the information you need to get started on your journey of working with essential oils.

ESSENTIAL OILS COVERED:
* Lavender- *Lavandula officinalis*
* Eucalyptus- *Eucalyptus globules*
* Rosemary- *Rosmarinus officinalis*
* Peppermint- *Mentha piperita*
* Tea Tree- *Melaleuca alternifolia*

EACH SECTION INCLUDES:
* Background Facts
* Therapeutic Properties
* Uses & Methods
* Uses for Emotions
* Dosage
* Cautions & Contra-Indications

FORMULAS:
Following each essential oil section, is a formula section for specific ways you can use the essential oil. Below are things to keep in mind when preparing your formulas.

* Gather all your supplies and materials before starting.

* Refer to carrier oil reference page to select the best suited carrier oil for your blend.

* Make sure your containers are clean. It is best to wash them with hot soapy water then allow them to air dry.

* When mixing essential oils, do not use metal utensils to mix, rather use a wooden spoon, glass stirrer or popsicle stick.

* Use clean <u>glass</u> containers when possible to store your blends. Small mason jars work well.

* If making a blend that will be used in the shower, use clean plastic bottles.

* PET & HDPE plastic bottles hold up to use with essential oils.

* Essential oils tend to disintegrate rubber, so be aware if you are using a bottle with a rubber bulb top, it will turn into a gooey mess after a short period of time.

* Be sure to label and date everything you make.

* Keep a record of your formula- I use an index card system to record my formulas so if I want to go back and make more, it is at my fingertips. Also it is a good idea to add notes to the card about how well you liked the formula, or whether you want to make any additions or deletions.

* Light, heat and oxygen will deteriorate you blends. Store your blend in the proper container, keep it in a cool place, away from direct light.

Materials and Supplies

Below is a list of materials and supplies to gather to work with your starter essential oils to create some of the formulas listed.

ESSENTIAL OILS
* Lavender- *Lavandula officinalis*
* Eucalyptus- *Eucalyptus globules*
* Rosemary- *Rosmarinus officinalis*
* Peppermint- *Mentha piperita*
* Tea Tree- *Melaleuca alternifolia*

CONTAINERS
* small mason jars
* small plastic bottles
* plastic spray bottles
* glass spray bottles
* 15 ml glass bottles
* foot bath tub or basin
* pocket sized spray mister

UTENSILS/BOWLS
* ceramic bowl
* glass bowl
* glass stirrers
* popsicle sticks
* wooden/ plastic spoons

CARRIER OILS CHOICES
* almond oil
* avocado oil
* calendula infused oil
* grapeseed oil
* jojoba oil
* olive oil
* peanut oil
* sesame oil
* sunflower oil
* wheat germ oil

INGREDIENTS/SUPPLIES

* Aloe Vera gel
* apple cider vinegar- natural
* aroma diffuser
* baking soda- pure, aluminum free
* band-aids
* bath towel
* beeswax pellets
* coconut milk
* cotton balls
* Dr. Bronner's Castile Soap
* dryer sheets- unscented
* Epsom salts
* fabric softener- natural
* Flax seed oil
* lemon juice- organic
* paper towels
* plastic wrap
* sea salt- coarse
* Stevia
* sugar- raw, organic
* vegetable glycerin
* vitamin E capsules
* vodka- high proof
* wash cloth
* water- distilled
* witch hazel
* white vinegar

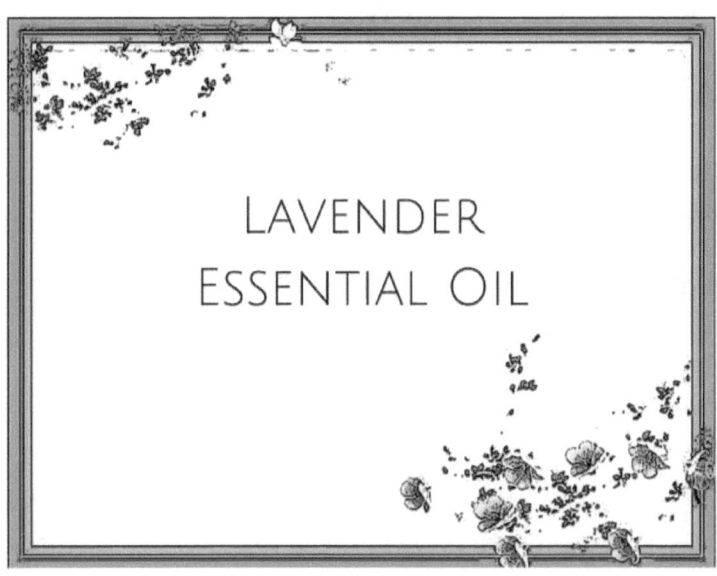

Lavender
Essential Oil

LAVENDER ESSENTIAL OIL

BACKGROUND FACTS

Latin Name: *Lavandula officinalis*
Common Name: Lavender
Extraction Method: Steam distillation of flowers
Color: Clear, with a hint of yellow
Aroma: Fresh, sweet, floral scent
Evaporation Rate: Top - Middle Note

THERAPEUTIC PROPERTIES

Analgesic
Anti-bacterial
Antidepressant
Antimicrobial
Antirheumatic
Antiseptic
Antispasmodic
Aromatic
Carminative
Emmenogogue
Hypotenstive
Insecticide
Nervine
Sedative
Stimulant
Stomachic
Vulnerary

USES AND METHODS

URINARY SYSTEM
<u>Uses</u>: Cystitis: <u>Methods</u>: sitz baths, baths, compresses, creams

RESPIRATORY SYSTEM:
<u>Uses</u>: asthma, bronchitis, coughs, halitosis, influenza, laryngitis, sinusitis, throat-infected. <u>Methods</u>: facial massage, inhalations, chest rubs, chest compresses, baths

MUSCULAR SYSTEM
<u>Uses</u>: lumbago, muscular aches and pains, rheumatism, sprains, joint paint. <u>Methods</u>: compresses, massage oils, baths

NERVOUS SYSTEM
<u>Uses</u>: depression, fainting, tension, headaches, hypertension, migraine, nervousness, stress, and insomnia. <u>Methods</u>: massage oils, compresses, baths, inhalations, herbal teas

REPRODUCTIVE SYSTEM
<u>Uses</u>: harmonize and regulate menstruation. <u>Methods</u>: compress, douche, sitz bath, massage

SKIN PROBLEMS
<u>Uses</u>: acne, sunburn, eczema, burns. <u>Methods</u>: lotions, creams, steaming, compress, baths

DIGESTIVE SYSTEM
<u>Uses</u>: cramps, colic, slow digestion, gas, indigestion, nausea, parasites. <u>Methods</u>: herbal teas, compress

LAVENDER FOR EMOTIONS

* Helps steady influences on the psyche
* Assists during times of indecisiveness
* Helpful during emotional conflict
* Has a balancing effect
* Helps calm strong or uncontrolled emotional states by bringing feeling under conscious control
* Helps steady extreme emotional states with a sense of rationality
* Good for depression

METHODS

Inhalers, diffuser, room sprays, baths, massage

DOSAGE

Adult: External: 5 - 10 drops in the bath
Inhalation: 2- 4 drops in 2 cups water
Massage Oil: 1 - 4 drops per TBSP carrier oil

CAUTIONS & CONTRA-INDICATIONS

* None known

FORMULAS USING LAVENDER

MIGRAINE
3-5 drops lavender essential oil
1 TSP carrier oil of your choice
   Blend essential oil with carrier oil. Massage onto affected area.

INSOMINA
A few drops lavender essential oil
   Add a few drops to a tissue or pillow case. Inhaling helps to
   soothe nerves, and relaxes the mind.

BUG BITE
1 drop lavender essential oil
cotton ball
   Add 1 drop of essential oil to cotton ball. Dab onto bug bite.
   Reduces swelling and pain.

FOOT SOAK
1 cup Epsom salts
10 drops lavender essential oil
Foot tub or basin
Warm water
   Fill basin with warm water. Stir in Epsom salts. Add essential
   oil. Soak feet 10 -15 minutes. Good for relaxing after a stressed
   day. Helpful before going to bed.

REMOVE SPLINTER
1 drop lavender essential oil
   Apply essential oil to splinter site. The splinter will slide out on
   its own.

MINOR BURNS
Lavender essential oil
Cold water
   Run burn under cold water for 10 minutes. Apply 1-2 drops to
   the affected area. Assists in the healing process. Also can be
   used for sunburn.

DETOX BATH
1 cup Epsom salts
1 cup baking soda
5-6 drops lavender essential oil
Warm bath water

Fill tub with warm bath water. Stir in Epsom salts and baking soda. Add essential oil drops. Mix well to disperse all ingredients. Make sure bathroom door is closed to keep the vapors in. Soak for 20 minutes for full benefits.

DRYER FRESHENER
Wash cloth
3-4 drops Lavender essential oil

To freshen clothes in the dryer, add a wash cloth with 3-4 drops of essential oil.

CUTS/SCRAPES
Band-aid
1-2 drops Lavender essential oil

Clean the cut or scrape. Add drops of essential oil to a band-aid before covering the affected area. Promotes healing and reduces scarring.

CARPET FRESHENER:
1 cup baking soda
5-6 drops lavender essential oil

Mix baking soda and essential oil. Sprinkle on rug. Let sit for 30 minutes. Vacuum as usual.

LINEN SPRAY
4 oz. glass spray bottle
2 TBS witch hazel
6 drops lavender essential oil
Distilled water

Add witch hazel and essential oil to spray bottle. Shake well for 1-2 minutes to blend well. Fill the remainder of the bottle with water. Shake again. Use as a linen spray. Add more drops of essential oil if you want a stronger scent.

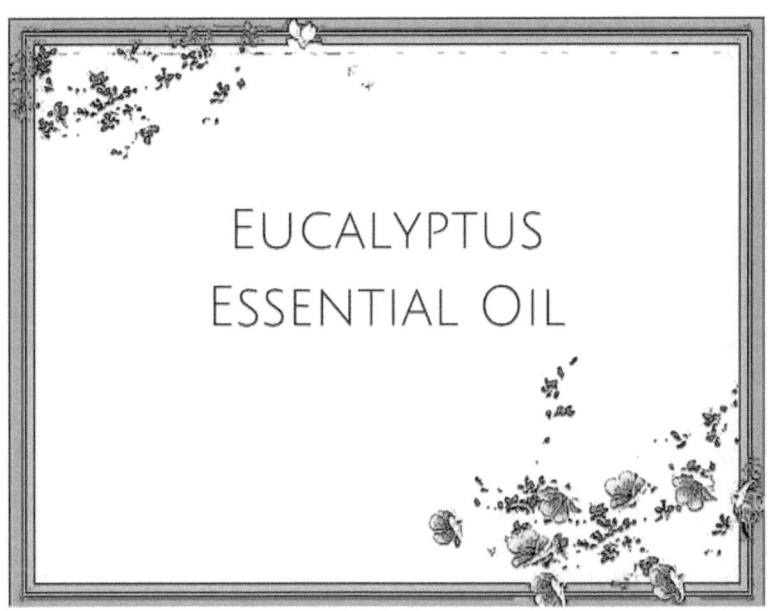

Eucalyptus
Essential Oil

EUCALYPTUS ESSENTIAL OIL

BACKGROUND FACTS

Latin Name: *Eucalyptus globules*
Common Name: Eucalyptus
Extraction Method: Steam distillation of leaves
Color: Colorless
Aroma: Distinct/crisp/camphoraceous/penetrating
Evaporation Rate: Top Note

THRAPEUTIC PROPERTIES

Analgesic
Anti-bacterial
Antifungal
Antineuralgic
Antirheumatic
Antiseptic
Antispasmodic
Antiviral
Decongestant
Deodorant
Diuretic
Expectorant
Febrifuge
Insecticide
Stimulant
Vulnerary

USES AND METHODS

RESPIRATORY SYSTEM
Uses: asthma, bronchitis, cough, infection, influenza, laryngitis, lung infections, pneumonia, sinusitis, sore throat. Methods: inhalations (except asthma), baths, chest and back rubs, diffuser, room sprays, nasal inhaler, chest compress, massage oil

SKIN PROBLEMS
Uses: abscesses, blisters, boils, bruises, burns, dandruff, deodorizer, herpes, insect bites, shingles, skin infections, stings, skin ulcers. Methods: compresses, baths, creams, salves, body spray diluted to 1-2 percent, massage oil

MUSCULAR SYSTEM
Uses: arthritis, muscle stiffness, rheumatism, general aches and pains. Methods: massage oils, baths

NERVOUS SYSTEM
Uses: headaches, migraine, neuralgia. Methods: massage oil, compresses, baths

IMMUNE SYSTEM
Uses: chicken pox, colds, infection, fever, influenza, measles, viral. Methods: room spray, herbal tea, baths

EUCALYPTUS FOR EMOTIONS

* Clears head of mental exhaustion and inability to concentrate
* Balances extreme moods
* Cools heated emotions when engaged in conflict-verbal, emotional, physical
* Creates feeling of space

METHODS

Inhalers, diffuser, room sprays, bath, massage

DOSAGE

Adult: 1 -3 drops
Bath: 5 - 10 drops
Inhalation: 2- 3 drops in 2 cups water
Massage Oil: 5 drops per TBSP carrier oil

CAUTIONS & CONTRA-INDICATIONS

* Do not apply to face or nose
* Do not exceed the stated dose
* Contra-indicated if there is a history of epilepsy, hypertension, gastrointestinal inflammation, liver complaints
* Do not use undiluted on skin
* Use with caution if taking medication-can reduce effects of medication

FORMULAS USING EUCALYPTUS

ACHY JOINTS
2 TBS Peanut oil
2-3 drops Eucalyptus essential oil
  Add essential oil to peanut oil, blend well. Massage into areas
  that are experiencing aches and pains.

BATH FOR COLD/CONGESTION
1 cup Epsom salts
6- 8 drops Eucalyptus essential oil
Tub filled with warm water
  Fill tub with the warmest water you can tolerate. Add Epsom
  salts, swish to mix well. Add essential oil, swish again to
  disperse. Close bathroom door so the vapors stay in the room.
  Breathe deeply. Soak for at least 20 minutes to get the full
  benefits. This bath also is helpful for achy muscles.

HAND DEGREASER
Small glass container
½ cup Sea salt
½ Epsom salt
5-6 drops Eucalyptus essential oil
  Mix salts together in glass jar. Blend in drops of essential oil.
  Cover jar with lid until ready to use. To use: wet hands and rub
  with a handful of your mixture.

SHOE ODOR
2 unscented dryer sheets
4 oz spray bottle
2 TSP witch hazel
6 drops Eucalyptus essential oil
Warm water
  Put witch hazel and essential oil in spray bottle. Shake a few
  minutes to blend well. Then fill the remainder of the bottle
  with warm water. Shake vigorously again. Spray dryer sheets
  with this blend. Put 1 dryer sheet into each shoe.

STICKER REMOVER

A few drops Eucalyptus essential oil
Paper towel or cloth
　　Add a few drops of essential oil to cloth or towel. Use to
　　remove stubborn stickers.

CHEST RUB

1 -2 TBS beeswax pellets
½ cup coconut oil or olive oil
10- 15 drops Eucalyptus essential oil
Small glass jar
　　Melt beeswax in a double boiler. Once the wax has melted,
　　add the coconut or olive oil. Heat slightly. Remove from heat.
　　Allow to cool a about a minute, then add essential oil drops.
　　Transfer to glass jar. Put lid on until ready to use. After a few
　　months, make a fresh batch. For children, use ½ the
　　amount of essential oil.

INVIGORATING SHOWER

5 drops Eucalyptus essential oil
　　Before entering the shower, add 5 drops of essential oil to the
　　shower floor. Shower as usual.

COLDS/CONGESTION

Bowl of boiling water
2-5 drops Eucalyptus essential oil
Bath towel
　　Fill bowl with boiling water. Add essential oil drops. Stir to
　　blend. Put your head over the bowl and inhale deeply, cover
　　with a towel to keep the vapors in.

ACNE

1 TBS natural Apple Cider Vinegar
2 drops Eucalyptus essential oil
Cotton ball
　　Blend apple cider vinegar and essential oil well. Dip cotton
　　ball in the blend, dab onto affected areas.

CAR FRESHENER

Cotton ball

1-2 drops Eucalyptus essential oil

Add 1-2 drops essential oil to cotton ball. Place in car. I like to put mine in the vent, so the air blows on it and disperses the vapors throughout the car. Replenish as needed. This is good when you have a cold or are feeling mentally or physically fatigued.

REMOVE INK FROM CLOTHES

Eucalyptus essential oil

Apply neat to ink stain on clothes.

ITCHY SCALP

1 TBS coconut oil

3-4 drops Eucalyptus essential oil

Plastic wrap

Mix coconut oil and essential oil together well. Massage into scalp. Wrap your head in plastic wrap. Leave on scalp a minimum of 30 minutes. Remove wrap and shampoo hair.

PERSONAL SPRITZ SPAY

Small purse size spray bottle

Witch hazel

Distilled water

5-10 drops Eucalyptus essential oil, depending on size of bottle

How much of the above ingredients you use, depends on the size of your spray bottle. Fill the bottle about an 1/8 way up with witch hazel. Add your essential oil drops, shake well to blend.

Fill the remainder of the bottle with distilled water. Use this spray to re-energize yourself when you need an energy lift. Shake well before use, spray 12 inches from face.

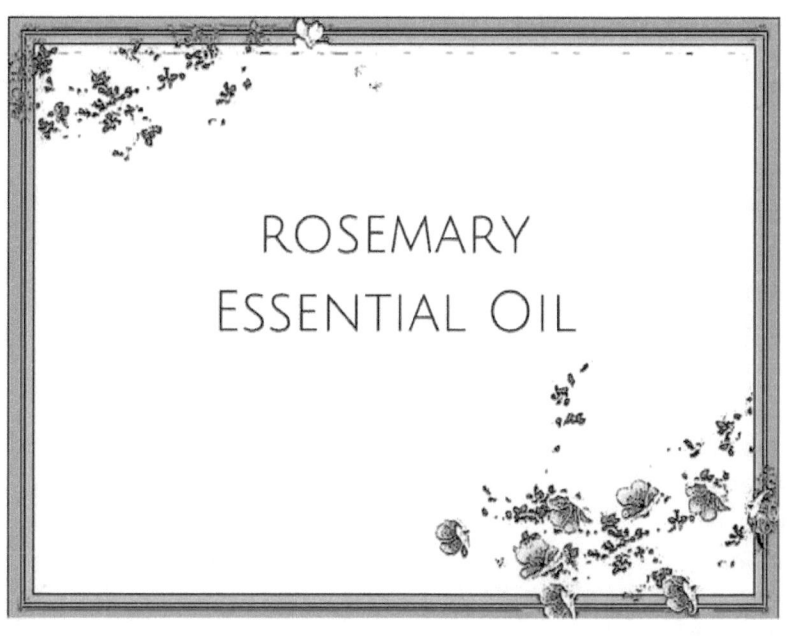

ROSEMARY
ESSENTIAL OIL

ROSEMARY ESSENTIAL OIL

BACKGROUND FACTS

Latin Name: *Rosmarinus officinalis*
Common Name: Rosemary
Extraction Method: Steam distillation of leaves
Color: Colorless
Aroma: Warm/sharp/refreshing/camphoraceous
Evaporation Rate: Middle Note

THERAPEUTIC PROPERTIES

Analgesic
Antiarthritic
Antibacterial
Antidepressant
Antifungal
Antineuralgic
Antiseptic
Antispasmodic
Astringent
Carminative
Digestive
Diuretic
Expectorant
Fungicidal
Insecticide
Hypertensive
Nervine
Restorative
Stomachic
Stimulant
Tonic
Vulnerary

USES & METHODS

RESPIRATORY SYSTEM
Uses: bronchitis, colds, coughs, influenza, respiratory infection, throat, tonsillitis, whooping cough. Methods: inhalations, chest and back rubs, diffuser, chest compresses, baths, nasal inhalers, room sprays, massage oil

MUSCULAR SYSTEM
Uses: muscle pains, rheumatism, gout, arthritis. Methods: massage oils, baths

NERVOUS SYSTEM
Uses: slow circulation, lack of concentration, dizziness, exhaustion, fainting, chronic fatigue, mental fatigue, headache, migraine, neuralgia. Methods: massage oil, compresses, baths, herbal teas

DIGESTIVE SYSTEM
Uses: constipation, diarrhea, gas, nausea. Methods: herbal tea, baths, massage, compresses

SKIN PROBLEMS
Uses: acne, burns, dandruff, dermatitis, oily hair, itching, lice, seborrhea, sores, swelling, wounds. Methods: lotions, salves, creams, ointments, compresses, massage oils, shampoos, conditioners

CIRCULATORY SYSTEM
Uses: gout, fluid retention, hypotension, palpitations. Methods: baths, herbal teas, massage oil

ROSEMARY FOR EMOTIONS

* Helps clear mind of confusion and doubt
* Stimulates sensitivity and helps increase creative thinking

METHODS

Inhalers, diffuser, room spray, baths, massage

DOSAGE

Adult: External 2-3 drops
Bath: 5 - 10 drops
Inhalation: 2- 3 drops in 2 cups water
Massage Oil: 5 drops per TBSP carrier oil

CAUTIONS & CONTRA-INDICATATIONS

* Skin patch test recommended
* Do not administer to children under 4
* Contra-indicated for first trimester of pregnancy
* Contra-indicated if there is a history of asthma, epilepsy,
   hypertension
* Do not use with homeopathic remedies or store near
   homeopathic remedies
* Do not use undiluted on skin

FORMULAS USING ROSEMARY

LEARNING/MEMORY
1 TBS Almond oil
2 drops Rosemary essential oil
  Blend almond oil and essential oil. Rub the massage oil onto
  your temples to help aid learning.

SINUS HEADACHE
1 drop Rosemary essential oil
1 drop Eucalyptus essential oil
2 drops Peppermint essential oil
2 drops Lavender
Aroma Diffuser
  Add the above drops into your aroma diffuser to help with a
  sinus headache. You can also use this ratio to mix into a 2TSP
  of carrier oil to make a massage blend that can be rubbed
  into the affected area.

CAR FRESHENER
Cotton ball
1-2 drops Rosemary essential oil
  Add 1-2 drops essential oil to cotton ball. Place in car. I like to
  put mine in the vent, so the air blows on it and disperses the
  vapors throughout the car. Replenish as needed. This is good
  when you have a long drive and need to stay alert and keep
  your mind sharp.

RESPIRATORY PROBLEMS
15 ml glass bottle
Sea Salt- coarse
5 drops Rosemary essential oils
  Fill the glass bottle with sea salt. Add drops of essential oil.
  Shake bottle vigorously to disperse the essential oil. Put top
  on bottle until ready to use. Inhale when needed. Shake
  before each use.

ACHY MUSCLES

Tub filled with hot water

1 cup Epsom salts

½ cup pure baking soda

½ cup sea salt

5-8 drops Rosemary essential oil

Fill tub with the warmest water you can tolerate. Add salts and baking soda, swish to mix well. Add essential oil, swish again to disperse. Close bathroom door so the vapors stay in the room. Breathe deeply. Soak for at least 20 minutes to get the full benefits.

BAGGY EYES

Small glass jar

4 TBS Aloe Vera gel

5 drops Rosemary essential oil

Mix ingredients into a clean mason jar, blend well. With a clean finger, carefully apply under baggy eyes. Keep jar in refrigerator when not in use.

IMPROVE CIRCULATION

2 oz. carrier oil of your choice

24 drops Rosemary essential oil

1 capsule vitamin E (optional)

Make a massage oil to increase circulation, especially if you experience tight muscles, that can impede blood flow, and often leads to symptoms such as numbness or cold hands and feet. Mix the carrier oil of your choice with the essential oil, shaking vigorously before use. In addition you can add 1 capsule of vitamin E oil to preserve the carrier oil. Massage the blend into the affected area.

SUGAR SCRUB FOR STRETCH MARKS
½ cup organic raw sugar
¼ cup organic coconut oil
1-2 TSP lemon juice
10 drops Rosemary essential oil
Small glass mason jar

Mix the sugar and coconut oil together. Add the lemon juice, adjust to get the right consistency. Add essential oil, blend well. Put the lid on the jar until ready to use. For stretch marks, rub affected areas with your sugar scrub in a circular motion. Rinse after application and follow up with a light layer of coconut oil to moisturize the skin. Use treatment 2 to 3 times per week.

MOSQUITO REPELLENT
Distilled water
20 drop Rosemary essential oil per ounce
Plastic spray bottle

Rosemary is a very effect mosquito repellent to use when outdoors. Fill your spray bottle with distilled water and add 20 drops of essential oil for each ounce of water. Shake well before spraying.

KITCHEN CLEANER
½ cup Distilled water
½ White vinegar
12 drops Rosemary essential oil
Spray bottle

Mix water and vinegar together in a spray bottle, then add essential oil. Shake vigorously to blend. Rosemary has antibacterial, antifungal and antiviral properties, which make it a good choice for use in cleaning the kitchen.

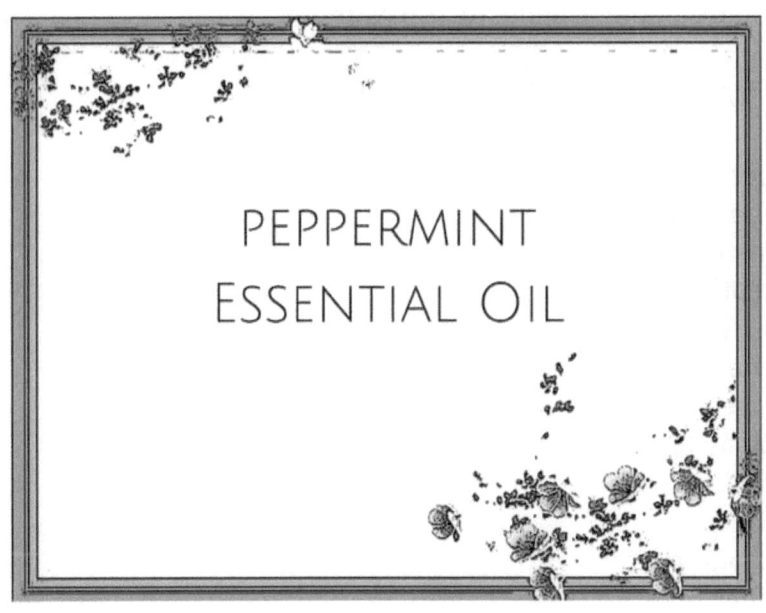

PEPPERMINT
ESSENTIAL OIL

PEPPERMINT ESSENTIAL OIL

BACKGROUND FACTS

Latin Name: *Mentha piperita*
Common Name: Peppermint
Extraction Method: Steam distillation of leaves
Color: Pale yellow or greenish
Aroma: Highly penetrating, grassy-minty odor
Evaporation Rate: Middle to Top Note

THERAPEUTIC PROPERTIES

Analgesic
Anti-inflammatory
Antimicrobial
Antiseptic
Antispasmodic
Antiviral
Astringent
Carminative
Cephalic
Cordial
Expectorant
Febrifuge
Heptic
Nervine
Vasoconstrictor
Vermifuge

USES & METHODS

URINARY
<u>Uses:</u> kidney tonic, menstrual cramps. <u>Methods:</u> sitz baths, baths, compresses, creams

RESPIRATORY
Uses: asthma, bronchitis, halitosis, laryngitis, sinusitis, spasmodic cough, dry cough, decongestant. Methods: inhalation (except asthma), chest rubs, compresses, baths, nasal inhalers, room sprays, vaporizers

MUSCULAR SYSTEM
Uses: muscle aches and pains, detoxification of connective tissue, rheumatism. Methods: compresses, creams, baths

NERVOUS SYSTEM
Uses: fainting, headaches, nervous stress, mental fatigue, migraine, vertigo. Methods: massage oil, compresses, baths, nasal inhalations

IMMUNE SYSTEM
Uses: colds, influenza, fevers. Methods: compresses, baths, herbal teas, massage, chest rub, room sprays, nasal inhalers

DIGESTIVE SYSTEM
Uses: cramps, colic, gas, nausea. Methods: herbal tea, honey water, massage

SKIN PROBLEMS
Uses: acne, dermatitis, ringworm, blackheads, toothache, detoxification, relieves itching, inflammation, softens skin, cools skin. Methods: lotions, creams. mouthwashes, compresses, massage oil, baths

PEPPERMINT FOR EMOTIONS

* Aids concentration and memory
* Stimulates the brain to think clearly
* Helps encourage a bright outlook
* Excellent for mental fatigue and depression
* Good remedy for shock

METHODS

Inhalers, diffusers, room sprays, baths, massage

DOSAGE

Adult: External 1-3 drops
Bath: 5 - 10 drops
Inhalation: 2- 3 drops in 2 cups water
Massage Oil: 5 drops per TBSP carrier oil

CAUTIONS & CONTRA-INDICATIONS

* Has been known to cause allergic reactions in the mouth, neck and throat when consumed in large doses
* Do not use in first trimester of pregnancy
* Do not use when breast feeding- may reduce milk production
* Do not use with children under 2
* Avoid in cases of heart disease, fever and epilepsy
* Avoid with homeopathic remedies
* Use externally for a limited time
* Do not use on damaged or sensitive skin
* Skin patch test recommended
* Avoid direct contact with the eyes

FORMULAS USING PEPPERMINT

MOUTHWASH
¾ cup water
¼ cup vodka
4 TSP liquid glycerin
1 TSP Aloe Vera gel
10 drops Peppermint essential oil
Glass jar

Mix all ingredients, store in a glass jar until ready to use. Shake before each use. Store in a cool place, away from direct light.

TOOTHPASTE
6 TBS Coconut oil
6 TBS Pure baking soda
15 drops Peppermint essential oil
1 TSP Stevia
Glass jar

Mix coconut oil and baking soda in glass jar. Add essential oil drops and mix well. Seal jar until ready for use. Coconut oil is solid at room temperature, so you may need to use a popsicle stick to spread the toothpaste onto your brush. Not recommended for children.

HEALTHY SHAMPOO
1/3 cup Dr. Bronner's Castile Soap
1/3 cup distilled water
1 TSP coconut oil
2 TSP baking soda
5 drops Peppermint essential oil
10 drops Lavender essential oil
Plastic bottle

Blend together all the ingredients in a bowl except essential oils. After everything is well mixed, add and blend your essential oils into the shampoo. Transfer to a plastic bottle to keep in the shower.

JOINT PAIN

1 oz. Carrier oil of your choice
15 drops Peppermint essential oil
Container: glass or plastic bottle

If you suffer from arthritis, this massage oil is helpful in combating joint pain. Mix your ingredients together and store in your container until ready for use. Shake well before each application.

BREATHE CLEAR NASAL INHALER

15 ml glass bottle
Coarse sea salt
2 drops Eucalyptus essential oil
2 drops Peppermint essential oil
1 drop Rosemary essential oil

Fill your glass bottle with coarse sea salt. Add each essential oil, shaking vigorously between each addition. Cap until ready for use. This is a great natural inhaler to use when you are all stuffed up and need to clear your sinuses. Shake before using, then breathe in deeply.

LICE TREATMENT

2 oz. Olive oil
15-20 drops Peppermint essential oil
Cotton balls
Plastic wrap

Mix olive oil and essential oil together. Using a cotton ball, dab the blend on your scalp. Once you have treated your entire head, cover completely with plastic wrap. Leave on overnight. Wash out in the morning.

FACE AND BODY WASH

2 oz. Dr. Bronner's Castile Soap
2 oz. Olive oil
2 oz. Vegetable glycerin
30 drops Tea Tree essential oil
5 drops Peppermint essential oil
5 drops Lavender essential oil
8 oz. Glass or plastic container

Mix all ingredients in a glass or ceramic bowl, then transfer to your container. Shake vigorously before each use. Store away from direct light and heat.

PET ODOR

3 ½ cups warm water
½ cup natural fabric softener
2 TSP baking soda
15 drops Peppermint essential oil
15 drops Tea Tree essential oil
Large spray bottle

In a bowl, mix water and baking soda together until well blended. Add fabric softener, mix well. Add essential oils. Stir until well mixed. Transfer to a spray bottle. Shake vigorously before each use.

EXFOLIATING SCRUB

½ cup natural cane sugar
2 TSP Coconut oil
1 TSP Flax seed oil
8 drops Peppermint essential oil
Glass mason jar

Mix all ingredients together in a glass mason jar for an exfoliating facial scrub.

CAR FRESHENER
Cotton ball
1-2 drops Peppermint essential oil
>Add 1-2 drops essential oil to cotton ball. Place in car. I like to put mine in the vent, so the air blows on it and disperses the vapors throughout the car. Replenish as needed. This is good for aiding alertness and concentration.

COOL A FEVER
2-3 drops Peppermint essential oil
Wet wash cloth
>Add a few drops essential oil to a wet wash cloth. Apply to forehead.

BREATH FRESHENER
Glass of warm water
1 drop Peppermint essential oil
>Place essential oil into water, stir. Swish your mouth with this blend. Spit out, rinse.

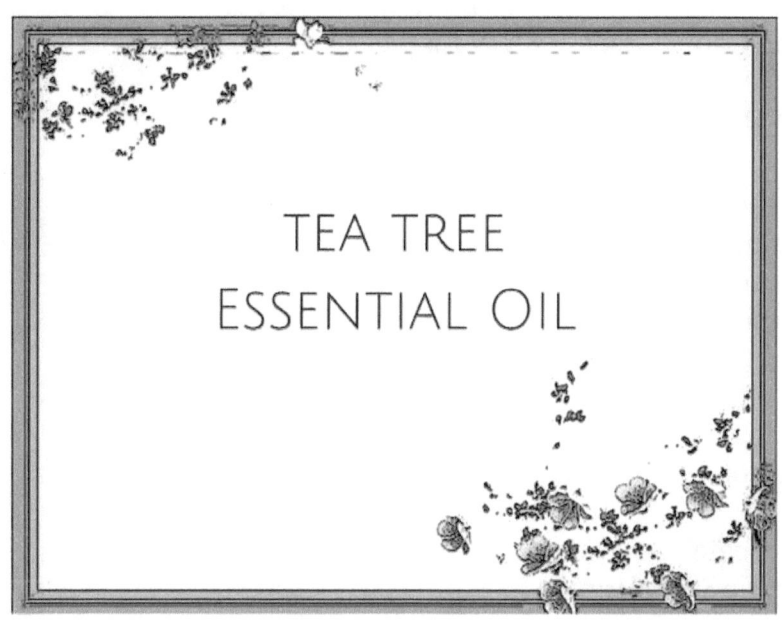

TEA TREE
ESSENTIAL OIL

TEA TREE ESSENTIAL OIL

BACKGROUND FACTS

Latin Name: *Melaleuca alternifolia*
Common Name: Australian Tea Tree
Extraction Method: Steam distillation of leaves
Color: White or pale yellow
Aroma: Fresh/sharp/pungent/camphoraceous
Evaporation Rate: Middle Note

THERAPEUTIC PROPERTIES

Antibacterial
Antifungal
Anti-inflammatory
Antimicrobial
Antiseptic
Antiviral
Deodorant
Expectorant
Germicidal
Insecticide
Immune Stimulant

USES & METHODS

URINARY SYSTEM
Uses: cystitis, urinary tract infection. Methods: sitz baths, baths, compresses, creams

RESPIRATORY SYSTEM
Uses: laryngitis, colds, coughs, influenza, sinusitis, lung infection, sinus congestion, throat-infected, throat-sore.
Methods: facial massage, inhalation, chest rubs, chest compresses, baths

REPRODUCTIVE SYSTEM
Uses: anal itching, genital itching, vaginal infection. Methods: tampon soaked with 1% solution, compresses, sitz bath, douche

SKIN PROBLEMS
Uses: abrasions, abscesses, acne, bed sores, blisters, boils, burns, cold sores, cracked skin, cuts, dandruff, body piercing-infected, eczema, fungal infections, gingivitis, gums-infected, insect bites, insect stings, muscular aches, nail infections, pimples, psoriasis, rashes, ringworm, skin-oily, sores, splinters, stings, sunburn, ticks, toothaches, ulcers-mouth, warts, wounds. Methods: steaming, massage, compresses, baths, creams, mouthwashes, rubbed on gums with diluted carrier oil

TEA TREE FOR EMOTIONS

* Clarifying
* Head clearing
* Cleanses imagination of disturbing thoughts

METHODS

Inhalers, diffusers, room sprays, baths, massage

DOSAGE

Adult: External: 1-3 drops
Bath: 5 - 10 drops
Inhalation: 2- 3 drops in 2 cups water
Massage Oil: 5 drops per TBSP carrier oil

CAUTIONS & CONTRA-INDICATIONS

* Skin patch test recommended for individuals with sensitive skin
* May cause skin irritation in rare cases

FORMULAS USING TEA TREE

ANTIBACTERIAL HAND CLEANER
1 TSP Aloe Vera gel
2 drops Tea Tree essential oil
   Mix together then clean hands.

GARGLE FOR SORE THROAT
Glass of warm water
2 TBS sea salt
1 drop Tea Tree essential oil
   Mix together, then gargle.

CLEAN CUTS & SCRAPES
1 TBS organic coconut oil
1 drop Tea Tree essential oil
   Clean cut with warm soapy water. Pat dry. Mix coconut oil
   and essential oil. Dab onto cut. Cover with a band-aid.
   Reapply as necessary.

ALL PURPOSE HOUSE CLEANER
Spray bottle
½ cup distilled white vinegar
¼ cup warm water
20 drops Tea Tree oil
   Mix all ingredients into spray bottle. Shake well. Use to clean
   and disinfect.

EAR INFECTION
1-2 drops Tea Tree essential oil
   Rub essential oil around base of the ear. Repeat every few
   hours as needed.

PIMPLES
1 drop Tea Tree essential oil
   Add essential oil to cotton ball. Dab on the problem area.
   Reapply as needed.

DISINFECT TOOTHBRUSH

1 drop Tea Tree essential oil
   Place neat onto toothbrush.

DANDRUFF

3 drops Tea Tree essential oil
2 TSP organic coconut oil
   Blend essential oil and coconut oil. Massage into head. Leave
   on at least 30 minutes. Then shampoo and wash out.

FACIAL SCRUB

½ cup organic coconut oil
¼ cup raw organic sugar
10 drops Tea Tree essential oil
   Combine coconut oil and sugar. Add drops of essential oil. Mix
   well. Store in a small glass jar.

SHAMPOO

Plastic bottle
¼ cup coconut milk
1/3 cup Dr. Bronner's Castile soap
1 TSP vitamin E oil or olive oil
10 drops Tea Tree essential oil
   Mix all ingredients in the plastic bottle. Shake well to blend.
   Use about 1TSP to shampoo hair. Shake bottle before each use.

RESOURCE: SUPPLIERS

FOR ESSENTIAL OILS

Aura Cacia
https://www.auracacia.com/

Frontier
http://www.bindependent.com/

Mountain Rose Herbs
https://www.mountainroseherbs.com/

NOW
https://www.nowfoods.com

Vitacost
http://www.vitacost.com/

Young Living
https://www.youngliving.com

BOTTLING

Container & Packaging Supply
https://www.containerandpackaging.com

SKS Bottling & Packaging
https://www.sks-bottle.com/

ABOUT
SEEDS FOR CHANGE WELLNESS

Hi!
The Anderson's here!

Seeds for Change Wellness is operated as a grassroots outreach program, in addition to our regular careers, providing educational programming and services to assist those who, like us, are striving for balance and harmony in their daily, often hectic lives.

We offer holistic classes and services in both our local community and out of state, with our main focus in the area of energy clearing of homes and properties. Our website, Seeds for Change Wellness, offers a wealth of information on a variety of topics in our article library on all things related to healthy living.

Scott & Susan

OTHER BOOKS FROM SEEDS FOR CHANGE WELLNESS

Breakfast Recipes: Grab & Go
ASIN: B01JKKOXDA

Dowsing: A Beginner's Pocket Guide
ASIN: B01JNR3G38

Essentially Yours: Aromatherapy Pocket Guide
ASIN: B01K3PH0SQ

FROM SUSAN ANDERSON

Going Deep: A Self-Discovery Journey
ISBN-13: 978-1537225470

FROM SUSAN ANDERSON & SLIM SPURLING

In the Mind of a Master
ISBN-10: 1475930720
ISBN-13: 978-1475930726